LOVING YOUR PREGNANT BODY

Dr. Talya Miron-Shatz and the Buddy&Soul Team

Pregnancy can feel like an alien invasion right inside your body! If you're finding it challenging to come to terms with some of the changes your body is going through, welcome to the club. In this book, you'll find helpful, research-based actions you can take to keep your self-esteem up and your unfounded expectations down this pregnancy, no matter what changes your body is going through.

There are three goals that we had in mind while creating this. We want you to:

- Accept your body regardless of its changes.

- Let go of critical thoughts, fears, and unrealistic expectations around your pregnant body.

- Appreciate the changes in your body as a part of the miracle of creating a new life.

Ah, pregnancy: the maternal glow, the beauty of creating a life, and of course…the growing belly! By now you know what to expect when you're expecting. You understand the changes to your appetite, chemistry, and emotions. You may even be the super-studious mother-to-be who has begun reading 'how to' child-rearing books. It's a bit in the future, but it's good to be prepared, right?

Right. Except that no one did much to prepare *you* for the out-of-body experience you seem to be having. Yet there's no two ways about it: that is *not* your body! Sure, the breasts have been super-sized, like you may have dreamed when you were reading preteen magazines, but that just adds to the creepy feeling that you are living in someone else's skin. Everything about you is different, from your hair down to your ankles— inasmuch as you can see them, that is. And it's not intuitive to love the way you look when you've gained weight in the most unlikely places.

But it's not impossible either.

Read on as we learn to build a more positive self-image, let go of critical thoughts about our pregnant bodies, and develop a newfound appreciation for everything our bodies are doing for ourselves and for our babies.

YOUR JOURNEY TO LOVING YOUR PREGNANT BODY

HOW TO USE THIS BOOK TO LOVE YOUR PREGNANT BODY

In this book you'll find ten great strategies for achieving the goals we listed above. You'll also find inspiring content and exercises you can engage with to help you practice loving your pregnant body.

You will get the most out of this book by going through the strategies and associated exercises one by one. Of course, you can also simply read it the whole way through. But we recommend using this book by going through it in order, watching the TED talks, and doing the exercises. We have found the best way to do the exercises is by dedicating a notebook as your course journal. If you're reading this book on a PC, feel free to create a text file and use that as your course journal. Or you could simply use a good ol' pen and paper to do the exercises. Either way, we recommend keeping some method of writing handy while you go through the exercises in this book to optimize what you get out of it.

To maximize your experience with the Buddy and Soul book, share your thoughts and insights with us on social media! Post pictures relating to your progress on Instagram and Twitter, tagging @Buddy_N_Soul, and Facebook @Buddy&Soul.   By sharing with us on social media, not only can you help others with their personal journeys, you can read about those facing similar challenges.

Direct message us YOUR story @Buddy_N_Soul on Instagram and be anonymously featured for a chance to **win a Buddy&Soul three month free membership**.

If you really want to go all the way, visit our website, BuddynSoul.com, and explore all that we have to offer beyond 'Loving Your Pregnancy Body'. In fact, we have three other books in the Pregnancy series that we think you might benefit from: Relationship Saver During Pregnancy, Sticking to Your Pregnancy Plan, and Acing the Fourth Trimester.

WHY I CREATED BUDDY&SOUL AND WHY I CREATED THIS BOOK

I'm Dr. Talya Miron-Shatz, CEO of Buddy&Soul, where Loving Your Pregnant Body and many more e-courses and books come from. I have a PhD in psychology and was very fortunate to do my post-doc at Princeton University with Nobel Laureate Daniel Kahneman. I've also taught at the Wharton Business School, University of Pennsylvania. Now I'm a professor at the Ono Academic College, and a visiting researcher at Cambridge University. I used to study happiness, and for a long time now, I've been studying medical decision making and helping organizations support people on their way to joy and health. One thing that struck me as unfair was that we were expecting people to change their life for good but weren't giving them the tools to do so. People deserve all the help they can get when breaking out of old patterns and moving their lives forward.

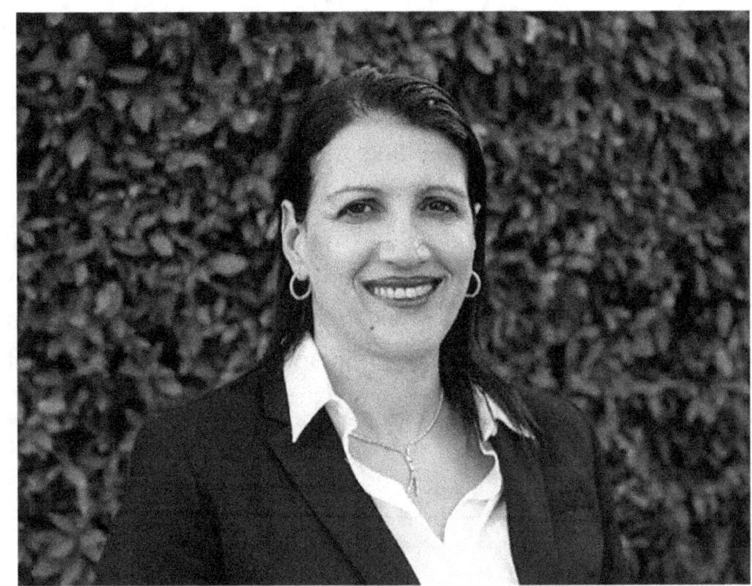

This is what Buddy&Soul does.

We support you in many ways by providing science-based actionable ways to sustain your body and mind. We help you sleep better, spark a change in your eating habits, and manage stress. We teach you how to create new habits and how to engage your willpower. We help you grow, claim your self-esteem, cultivate authenticity, reframe your life story, achieve your goals and so much more. Including Loving Your Pregnant Body. Which, being a woman, I particularly appreciate.

We created unique course clusters for people dealing with specific challenges: students, patients, and pregnant women.

Everything you need to change your life for good.

I want to hear from YOU! Please feel free to send me an email with your thoughts, suggestions, and feedback regarding this book to talya@buddynsoul.com. I would love to hear what you think about this book and how it helped you with loving your pregnant body. Your feedback is extremely valuable and will allow us to help more individuals, like yourself, to obtain the necessary tools and support needed to change their lives for good.

8 Benefits of learning to love your pregnant body

Learning to love your pregnant body is an incredible gift you can give yourself and your baby. Here are some benefits of investing in better body image during pregnancy.

1. Studies demonstrate that positive body image during pregnancy positively impacts both your own wellbeing and your baby's.
2. Letting go of thoughts about how your body *should* look is great preparation for parenthood, when you'll have to let go of all sorts of expectations of how things *should* be.
3. Why waste 9 months of your life hating the way you look? Time hatin' is time wastin'.
4. Your body will look the same whether you hate it or love it. Might as well love it.
5. Loving your pregnant body will carry over into loving your post-birth body.

Add your own ideas:

6. ____

7. ____

8. ____

Good body image and pregnancy just don't jive

Loving your pregnant body is a great idea, but it's not more than that. Here's why it doesn't spill over into the realm of reality.

For:

1. Good body image means slim. At least that's what we've been made to believe. That doesn't fit with pregnant.
2. When's the last time you saw an ad, or any media image for that matter, featuring a pregnant model when it wasn't for pitching a maternity product? Never. Because pregnant doesn't sell.
3. Pregnancy is not meant to be a time to think about your body. It's a time to think about your baby.

Add your own:

4. ____

Against:

1. Good body image is good body image, all the time: It doesn't matter if you're pregnant, trying to conceive, post-partum, or have no thoughts of pregnancy at all – any old time is fair game for positive body image!
2. Media images don't determine the way I feel about my body. At least, they shouldn't.
3. I love the way I look when I'm pregnant! That's why they call it a pregnancy glow.

Add your own:

4. ____

STRATEGY 1: Gain some weight... and love it!

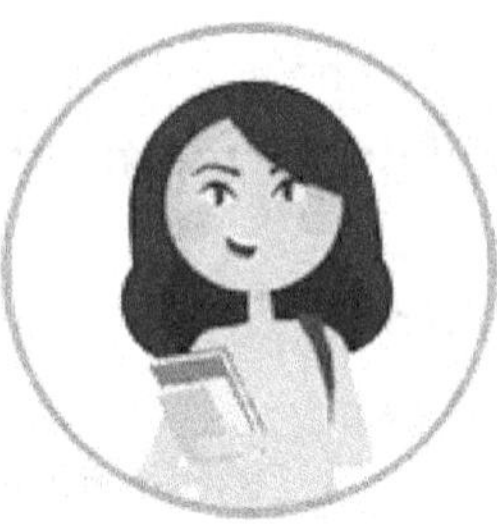

It is great that you have decided to begin the journey of Loving Your Pregnant Body. Each session within this book consists of a warm-up followed by a hands-on component where you'll learn a new skill or idea and have a chance to start putting it into action.

We're going to start the Loving Your Pregnant Body course by taking a look at how women really feel about their pregnant bodies, as opposed to what the media tell us to feel.

Watch 'Picturing pregnancy' presented by Meredith Nash at TEDxHobart on YouTube.

Sociologist Meredith Nash explains her research on how women experience their own pregnancies. To get to the bottom of it, she gave pregnant Tasmanian women digital cameras and asked them to photograph whatever they felt best captured their lives and experiences. Two years and 2000 photographs later, she explains why these pictures invite new possibilities for thinking about pregnant body image.

We think you'll find that the more you put into the course, the more you'll get out of it. So, take full advantage of this book and find your place in a community of people facing similar challenges.

The invitation I got to think differently about my pregnant body

Most of us have pre-conceived notions about pregnancy and body image, perhaps not all of them positive. Being pregnant offers you the opportunity to re-think some of those ideas. Spend a few minutes jotting down what sparked a change in the way you view your pregnant body in your journal.

Direct message us YOUR story @Buddy_N_Soul on Instagram and be anonymously featured for a chance to **win a Buddy&Soul three month free membership**.

DRIVING THE MESSAGE HOME

Pregnant women will often equate themselves to very large mammals. An elephant is a popular one. Or a whale. Some will be more creative and say, "I am the size of a delivery truck" or "a jumbo jet." Not all women fall into this camp, but if you find yourself coming up with these metaphors, and resenting them, it's time to get acquainted with some facts.

Fact number one: your body will grow. That's good, expected, and necessary.
And, assuming you're gaining properly, it's the healthiest thing for both mom and baby.

While pregnancy weight gain might not have been viewed as demonic in the past, Australian-based sociologist Meredith Nash (2012) explains there has been a cultural shift in past years. In her words, "women in the West now feel enormous pressure to conform to unachievable standards of (non-pregnant) feminine beauty" (*Making 'Postmodern' Mothers*, p. 35).

Why? What's the big deal with getting large anyway?

Fact number two: for most women who fear pregnancy weight gain, it's about more than just the extra pounds.

In the book, Nash further explains that fear of 'getting fat' has a strong psychological component too. In the research, she explains, "'Fat' was viewed… as more than just a substance to be shed post-birth; it was a frame of mind that this group of women often relied upon when they were feeling as though their bodies were out of control" (p. 40).

But perhaps most interestingly, research also found a discrepancy between how women viewed their own pregnancy weight gain versus how they understood pregnancy weight gain in general. In a study called *"Bumps and Boobs:" Fatness and Women's Experiences of Pregnancy*, researcher Sarah Earle found that women seemed willing to accept that weight gain is normal during pregnancy. However, when it came to their *own* pregnant bodies, weight gain was wholly unacceptable.

Accepting healthy weight gain as part of *your own* pregnancy and recognizing where your fears around weight gain are coming from are the very first steps towards loving and properly nourishing your pregnant body. And your baby too!

EXERCISE

Write your own body a permission slip stating, in the kindest terms possible, that you allow it to do what it's already doing – change, grow, and create space to nurture your growing baby.

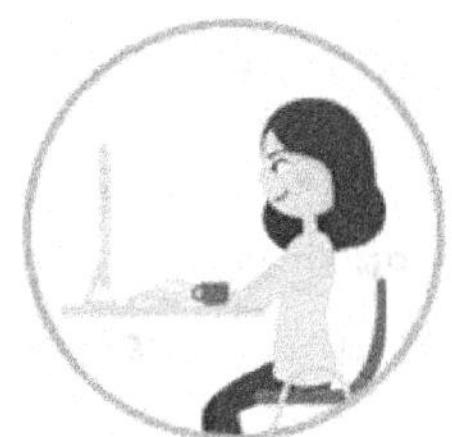

Include a reassuring sentence or two about why healthy weight gain need not scare you, nor make you feel at a loss for control.

TIPS

Tip 1: You might know in your *head* that you need to gain weight this pregnancy, but getting it down in writing will help move the knowledge from your head to your gut, no pun intended.

Tip 2: For more on self-acceptance and self-compassion, check out our Declutter Your Mind course. 

Tip 3: If you find you are pretty open to your body's changes during pregnancy, good for you! However, if you find there is some hesitation there, ask yourself whether it's the physical pounds you're afraid of, or if there may be something deeper lurking beneath the surface.

Tip 4: Help yourself remember! Take a picture and use your permission slip as the background for your phone or computer. Alternatively, take the physical permission slip and hang it somewhere prominent, like on your fridge or bathroom mirror.

7 TIPS FOR ACCEPTING YOUR PREGNANT BODY WITHOUT JUDGEMENT

It can be so hard to feel good about your body when it's changing at a pace so rapid and in a manner so foreign that you're unsure it's really you from the neck down. Here are some tips that can help you accept the changes in your pregnant body without judgment.

1. Remind yourself that you are not always in full control of your body but that you *are* in control of how you feel about the way you look.
2. Train yourself to think positively. For every negative thought you have about your pregnant body, make yourself come up with at least two positive thoughts.
3. Focus on the features of your pregnant body that you do love – whether that means those that haven't changed much, or those that have changed in ways that make you say "ooh la la!"
4. Reprogram your mind to embrace healthy weight gain (within the range your doctor deems okay). It means you are doing something right for your body and your baby!

Do you have any tips to add?

5. ____

6. ____

7. ____

IS BEFRIENDING MY PREGNANT BODY A USELESS GOAL?

If my pregnant body is not my permanent body, and this time period will be over in nine short months max, why bother putting all that effort into trying to love and accept my pregnant body? Seems like such a waste.

For:

1. I'd rather spend my limited energy focusing on other things like improving my relationship with my partner before the baby comes.
2. Why bother? It'll be over before I know it.
3. Pregnancy is not a time for befriending my body. It's a time for just not thinking about it, between doctor's appointments, that is.

Why do you think body positivity during pregnancy is a useless goal?

4. ____

Against:

1. We should always befriend our bodies. I want to feel good in the skin I'm in whether I'm pregnant or not.
2. How I feel about my body right now impacts my baby. I couldn't imagine a more important reason to befriend my pregnant body.
3. I consider it a challenge. And I always love a good challenge.
4. Pregnancy is the easiest time for me to befriend my body. It helps me accept my weight gain when I know there's a good reason for it.

What would be a benefit of having a positive body image while pregnant

5. ____

HOW I CHANGED MY APPROACH TO PREGNANCY WEIGHT GAIN

A lot of women anticipate gaining weight with dread, but it's a healthy part of pregnancy. If you've been able to take a positive angle on your weight gain write down some of your ideas in your journal.

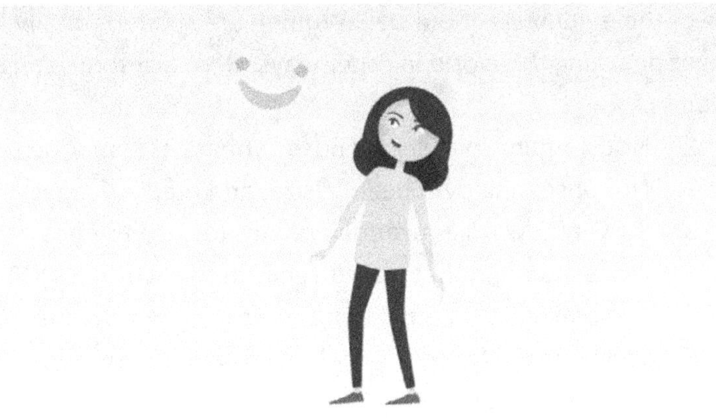

Little girls grow up hearing both implicitly and explicitly that the most important attribute they can strive for is beauty. A media culture that focuses on denigrating women who fail to meet the beauty standard turns women against women and sends men the message that evaluative commentary on appearance is fair game. The chronic focus on beauty directs cognitive, financial, and emotional resources away from other, more important goals.

When you're pregnant, that emphasis on cut-throat beauty can translate into a disproportionate emphasis on what your pregnant body *looks like* instead of on the function it's serving, i.e. growing a baby.

Watch 'An Epidemic of Beauty Sickness' by Renee Engeln at TEDxUConn on YouTube!

In her TED talk Dr. Renee Engeln, a psychologist and body image researcher at Northwestern University, considers whether there is hope for treating the epidemic of beauty sickness. She considers what it might be like to live in a world where women spend less time in front of the mirror and more time changing the world.

As you watch, think about the role beauty sickness plays in how you're relating to your body during pregnancy.

12 Tips for overcoming 'beauty sickness'

In her TEDx Talk, *An Epidemic of Beauty Sickness*, Dr. Renee Engeln speaks about 'beauty sickness' as one of the epidemics of our day. Women are so emotionally invested in their looks that they are no longer engaging the world in other ways. Here are some suggestions for overcoming this 'beauty sickness.'

1. Not standing in a 'skinny pose' whenever someone takes out a camera.
2. Not obsessing over beauty, size, and media images.
3. Striving toward education and not toward thinness.
4. Understanding that our currency in this world is NOT our appearance.
5. Not making it our goal to fit into a double zero size after birth, or ever.
6. Trying not to think of your body as a thing for others to look at all the time.
7. Limiting mirror time.
8. Not trash-talking our body, nor anyone else's for that matter.
9. Complimenting other women's admirable qualities rather than their looks.

Add your own:

10. ____

11. ____

12. ____

DRIVING THE MESSAGE HOME

Clothes are more than merely functional. Each time we choose a color, cut, or length, we make a statement about ourselves. We broadcast not only our tastes and preferences, but also our values and social allegiances. In short, clothes are part and parcel of the façade we bring to the world.
Now, we've all heard the tired advice to "dress for the job you want, not the job you have." In a work environment, that makes sense (unless you're a construction worker who dreams of being a showgirl, in which case, don't). But when you're dealing with your body image, unrealistic expectations have the power to be more harmful than helpful.

In a paper called *Pregnancy and Body Image: Analysis of Clothing Functions of Maternity Wear*, researchers Sohn and Bye discovered a subtle but fascinating connection between body image and maternity wear. Pregnant women with positive body image opted for maternity clothing as their bodies grew, while those with negative body image tended not to.

But why?

Well, it seems that **pregnant women who feel good about their bodies look for clothing that offers comfort and assurance**. In contrast, those who feel uncomfortable in their skin look for clothing that will hide their bodies.

(As a hopeful aside, the researchers actually found that the majority of pregnant women they surveyed did have pretty positive body image. Ten points for loving our pregnant bodies!)

If it's true that body image determines the wardrobe choices we make, then surely it can work the other way too – we can boost our body image by choosing appropriate clothing.

Removing the temptation of the form-fitting tops, pants, and dresses of your pre-pregnancy days will enable you to make better wardrobe choices as your pregnancy continues.

Sure, you may still be able to squeeze into some of your favorites during the first few weeks (with exponential difficulty starting week 15 or so), but the first time that zipper betrays you — because you somehow gained weight on your back — you may find yourself utterly devastated. Why set yourself up for that?

By allowing yourself to wear things like empire waists or elastic-banded slacks from earlier on, you'll ensure that the extra weight and shift in your body shape don't hit you one morning like a hammer to the face.

Of course, this can be done gradually. You needn't part with all your favorite pieces from week one. Just remember that beautifully designed maternity clothes are there for a reason, and there's no shame in wearing them, and no particular honor in wearing your uncomfortable regular clothes all the way up to your third trimester either.

EXERCISE

Spend about a couple of minutes **looking for images of pretty maternity wear that you think could be flattering on you.** Screenshot a picture of the best item you found. Think of it as online window shopping! Share your favorite image with the Buddy and Soul community! Tag us on Instagram and Twitter @Buddy_N_Soul, using the #BuddynSoulExpecting. By sharing with us on social media, not only can you help others with their personal journeys, you can read about those facing similar challenges.

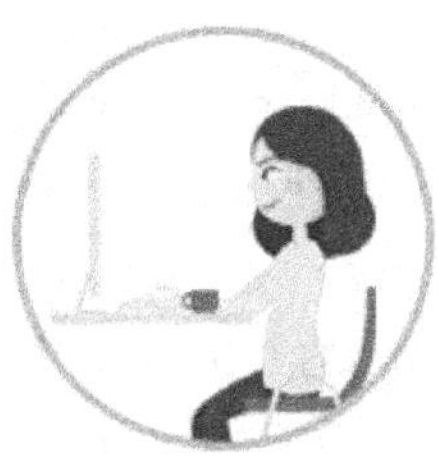

TIPS

Tip 1: When it comes to maternity wear, you can have some fun by considering styles you would never dream of donning in your normal, non-pregnant, state. It's a great opportunity to try out a new look.

Tip 2: Having trouble rocking a look you're not used to? Check out our Cultivating Authenticity course 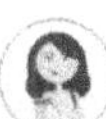 for more on bridging the gap between how you feel on the inside and what you present to the world.

11 Not-so-obvious reasons to invest in maternity wear

While it might be possible to squeeze into your regular stuff, here are some compelling reasons to opt for maternity clothing, whether bought, borrowed, or home-made.

1. You'll have more space to breathe, literally, since maternity clothes are designed with your growing belly in mind.
2. It's convenient. You won't have to sort through what no longer fits.
3. For the shoppers among us – another excuse to hit the mall!
4. Fact is, you're having a baby. Wearing maternity wear is another way to get the news out.
5. Maternity wear helps keep you covered. No more pulling your shirt down to meet your waist or leaving your jeans unbuttoned and hoping that no one will notice.
6. Larger-sized clothing or old baggy t-shirts are just less flattering than specially-tailored maternity clothes.
7. You deserve to feel pretty when you're pregnant. Even if it's temporary!
8. After the baby is born, it takes a little while to get back into shape again. You'll be happy you have some stretchy stuff in your wardrobe.

Can you think of any other reasons?

9. ____

10. ____

11. ____

Even the best maternity clothes can't make me love my body.

When I don't feel good about myself inside, fancying up the externals doesn't do a thing. Why in the world should I invest in a wardrobe change when I know it's all a big show?

For:

1. I don't recognize my pregnant body. Wearing my familiar clothes at least gives me some semblance of control.
2. Maternity clothes be like: whoa belly! While I would love to accept my body during pregnancy, I do *not* want my belly to be gawked at like a celebrity on vacation.
3. I think what will help me love my body is giving birth already. Wardrobe changes won't make much of a difference, I'm afraid.

Add your own ideas:

4. ____

Against:

1. Good maternity clothes are made to measure! They are flattering, feminine, and gorgeous.
2. Denial. That's what's keeping me in my Levis that no longer fit by any stretch of the imagination. I gotta accept that my body is now different, and own it. Because hey, I'm pregnant!
3. Who said that maternity clothes need to be some major investment? If I borrow, swap, or buy second-hand, I'll be much more willing to go there.

What is another reason why maternity clothes would help you to love your new body?

4. ____

I changed how I dressed during pregnancy and here's why

Generally speaking, there are two types of pregnant women – those who are itching to put on maternity wear, and those who swear they'll never let go of their skinny jeans. What made you decide to make the change and what difference did it make? Use your journal to express what changed your mind.

Direct message us YOUR story @Buddy_N_Soul on Instagram and be anonymously featured for a chance to **win a Buddy&Soul three month free membership**.

STRATEGY 3: Get real about your pregnancy role models

About 10,000 people a month Google the phrase "Am I ugly?" or look to social media to form their views of their own self-image. Self-esteem waxes and wanes instantaneously based on the number of likes people get on a selfie!

Pregnancy has the ability to exacerbate an already rocky relationship with one's body. And turning to the wrong role models doesn't help. Understanding who we are looking towards as our role models can directly influence our wellbeing and happiness during pregnancy.

In a deeply unsettling talk, self-esteem advocate Meaghan Ramsey of the Dove Self-Esteem Project walks us through the surprising impacts of low body image, from lower grade point averages to greater risk-taking with drugs and alcohol. Finally, she shares some take-homes about how we can change this reality and reclaim our rights to how we feel about our bodies.

Watch 'Why Thinking You're Ugly is Bad for You' presented by Meaghan Ramsey on www.ted.com.

An important watch for any pregnant woman for sure!

Actually, yes. Social media determines how beautiful I am.

In today's day and age, life is all about your online persona. If you don't make it there, you don't really make it anywhere. So, let's drop the illusions and call a spade a spade: my beauty *is* determined by what my online social network thinks of me.

For:

1. If you want to make it in life, you have to make it online.
2. Online, I can get hundreds of opinions at the drop of a hat. That's way more valid than the few opinions of my handful of friends.
3. Online relationships aren't censored. If I really want to know if I'm pretty, I have to expose myself to the brutal honesty of the masses.

Add your own idea:

4. ____

Against:

1. There is no culture of sensitivity or empathy online. Often, people are just brutal and critical for the sake of being brutal and critical. Their opinions really bear no weight, as far as I'm concerned.
   (Plus: Check out our Defining Your Identity course)
2. People online don't know me. How could they possibly be fit to judge my self-image? You need to know the whole package!
3. Studies are showing the opposite; that social media make you feel bad about yourself. It doesn't even seem to matter if it's true or not, because it's about how you feel and not about what you actually look like.

Add your own idea:

4. ____

DRIVING THE MESSAGE HOME

The big wide world has its way of broadcasting on loudspeaker the message that we're just not enough. When it comes to our pregnant bodies, that can mean anything from not graceful enough, to not sexy enough, to not carrying our baby weight beautifully enough. The list goes on.

And social media doesn't do much to quell our insecurities. Scan your newsfeed and you'll see what I mean. Most images set standards that are beyond impossible to achieve.

Post-birth women stepping out of the hospital in high heels and jeggings, which they wore all the way to their 26th week, by the way. Pregnancy being given the cutesy title of 'a bump,' as if a pregnant body were nothing more than a small round ball atop an otherwise 2-dimensional figure.

If you look that way naturally and without it costing your health or your baby's, great! But if this isn't exactly what you see or how you feel when you look in the mirror, that's fine too. In fact, it's more than fine. Because **no matter how our pregnant bodies look, we *are* enough.**

It's time to hit the pause button and stop holding ourselves to outlandish standards.

Instead of turning to those impossibly fly, one-in-a-million pregnant ladies as our compass, let's start turning to real-time women we know. Our mothers, friends, sisters, coworkers, and neighbors can offer far more honest representations of how a pregnancy looks and feels.

Real women, with real pregnancies, not only provide a more truthful frame of reference, but are actually more influential to our perceptions (*Making 'Postmodern' Mothers*, p. 7).

While you could still feel inadequate in comparison to some of the real-life pregnant women you know, the idea here is to choose someone with whom you can check out your story.

For instance, if your sister looked like the Energizer bunny throughout her pregnancy and you're feeling more like a retired maze rat, ask her about it. Ask her if she really felt as energetic as she looked, and if so, if there was anything she did to boost her energy. You can also ask if there were challenging aspects of her pregnancy that you might not have known about, since photos of bathroom accidents, regurgitated lunches, and workplace pass-outs probably didn't make the social media cut.

As you check out your perceptions of other women's pregnancies, you'll probably find that *no one* has a picture-perfect pregnancy. Sure, some have it easier and some have it harder, but even among those who seem to sail right through all three trimesters, there's usually more to the pregnancy than meets the public eye.

Go ahead, find yourself a real-life role model, and start getting real about your pregnancy expectations.

EXERCISE

Step 1: **Identify your pregnancy role model** — someone whose attitude towards pregnancy and her pregnant body inspires you. Whether she's your neighbor, sister, coworker, or best friend, write her name down in the space provided.

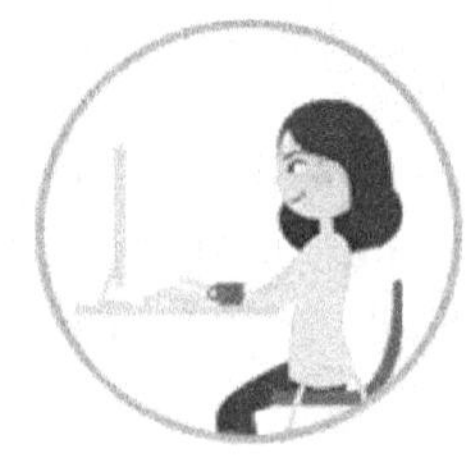

Step 2: You're Ellen, or Oprah, or some other fabulous talk show host. Your guest today is none other than the role model you just identified in Step 1.

Take a moment to imagine the back-and-forth that occurs during the interview. What do you ask? What does she respond?

Afterwards, jot down any insights or real-time questions you'd like to ask.

TIPS

Tip 1: Learn more about upping your internal sense of self-worth in a world where we're told that we're never good enough. Check out our Claim Your Self-Esteem course.

Tip 2: Even if you're planning to speak to someone you don't know very well, no need to make it a grill session. Lighten up and imagine it more along the lines of a conversation with an old friend.

Tip 3: No real-life role model? No problem. It's just as effective to imagine a conversation with an inspiring fictional character from a movie or book.

11 Expectations I will not have of my pregnant body

Our unmet expectations can be the culprits of negative feelings we harbor towards our pregnant bodies. If we didn't expect to look a certain way, we'd probably only feel good about our bodies. Here are some expectations that we recommend ***not*** having of your body this pregnancy!

1. I will not expect to look like a magazine image during any month of my pregnancy.
2. I will not expect my tummy or my body to look like anyone else's did.
3. I will not expect my boobs to go up in size. Or down in size. Or heck, I just won't expect anything from them!
4. I will not expect to lose my baby weight a week after I've given birth.
5. I will not expect to only gain only the exact weight of my baby. There is a certain amount of healthy extra weight needed for making a baby, not to mention the placenta, the amniotic fluid, and all that other fun stuff that joins the party.
6. I will not expect to move around with the same agility I could when I was not pregnant.
7. I will not expect my libido levels to remain unchanged with all those wonky hormones floating around.
8. I will not demand perfection from my body. Pregnancy is not a time for body perfection, and truthfully neither is any other time.

Do you have any other suggestions? Write them down!

9. ____

10. ____

11. ____

A pregnancy role model will just make me feel inadequate

When I compare myself to people around me, I feel worse. It doesn't matter if I'm comparing myself to my neighbor or to Demi Moore on the cover of Vanity Fair. The bottom line is that a pregnancy role model will just give me another opportunity to compare and feel worse about my pregnant body.

For:

1. Other people always seem to have things all figured out; I always seem to fall short. Why bother looking for a pregnancy role model who will exacerbate all my feelings of inadequacy and insecurity?
2. I'm not quite sure how another woman can be a role model for me and yet give me the space I need to figure it out on my own at the same time.
3. Comparisons are never fruitful. My chances of positive self-image are exponentially higher when I turn inwards instead.

Add your own reason:

4. ____

Against:

1. If I choose a pregnancy role model who is supportive and kind, I can check out all my insecurities with her. Does she *really* have it all figured out? And if so, what's her secret!?
2. I've experienced so many changes in this pregnancy and I need reassurance. Talking to a real woman who's been there and done that could really help me.
3. Feeling inadequate is just a feeling. If I could put that feeling aside, I would be open to learning from someone else's experience.

How would having a pregnancy role model help you?

4. ____

The amazing role model who revamped my view of pregnancy

We're drowning in information, especially online, but often we're lacking clarity. Having a role model for pregnancy can be a lifesaver. Take a few moments to write about *your* pregnancy role model and the wisdom that she shared with you in your journal.

Direct message us YOUR story @Buddy_N_Soul on Instagram and be anonymously featured for a chance to **win a Buddy&Soul three month free membership**. Share the wisdom!

<u>STRATEGY 4: Remember you're growing a baby in there!</u>

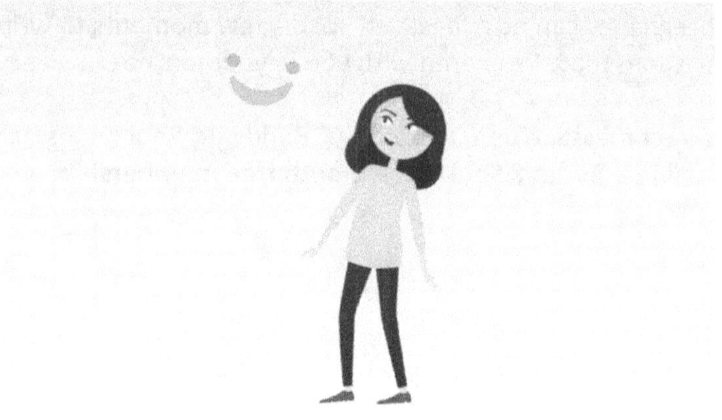

Jade Beall is a photographer from Tucson, AZ who seeks to empower women through photography. She launched her project for a book containing nude photos of mothers and pregnant women without retouching of any kind called "Bodies of Mothers" and became an instant sensation worldwide.

Beall wants to redefine human beauty by showing the world that beauty comes in all sizes, shapes, colors, with all kinds of stretch marks and imperfections. No Photoshop allowed.

Watch 'Bodies of Mothers' presented by Jade Beall at TEDxPitic on YouTube.

As you watch, try to internalize her positive message, that the body and love of a mother surpass all boundaries.

What media messages do you find helpful during pregnancy?

The media messages we are inundated with can really affect how we feel about our pregnant bodies. Which of these media messages do you wish you'd hear more often during pregnancy?

1. The dangers of smoking and drinking while pregnant.
2. Nurturing yourself helps you nurture your baby.
3. Weight gain during pregnancy is healthy and recommended.
4. That pregnancy is cross-cultural, including models and Hollywood stars.
5. There are no media messages that make me feel good about my pregnant body!

Are there any other media messages that you would find helpful?

6. ____

7. ____

8. ____

DRIVING THE MESSAGE HOME

When asked about your body during pregnancy, do you tend to focus on *either* yourself *or* on your growing baby?

Most women do.

And yet, the truth is that your body is currently pulling the old 2-for-1: one body serving the needs of two.

Rather than thinking about this as a tug of war, you'll foster healthier, more positive body image if you embrace your body's dual function. Just as pregnancy is about both mom and babe, so is your pregnant body. It's not one or the other.

Even the science agrees. One team of researchers found that women who embraced the duality of the pregnant body viewed their own physical changes more positively. They saw changes as indicators of their babies' health and growth and a sign of their adequacy as mothers. In other words, these women saw their growing bellies as a part of the bigger picture of creating a healthy baby. It was physical proof that their babies were growing and were one step closer to being in their arms.

That's not to say that you should take it to the other extreme and view yourself or your own needs as null and void. It's your body, indeed. But it's also your baby's home for nine months. It's almost like you're renting out space in your body, and the two of you gotta negotiate some way to make it work. Remembering that there is a baby growing inside of you, and that you are not redistributing your body's alignment for the sheer fun of it, can make all the difference in how you view your pregnant body. A conscious awareness of the miracle inside you can translate into greater respect and appreciation for your body, and, by extension, improved body image.

By simply allowing your pregnant body to 'do its thing,' you are literally creating a space for another human being in this world. And that's definitely something worth appreciating!

Beyond that, it also gives you a nice comeback if anyone calls and asks what you're up to:

"I'm gestating."

Beat THAT!

EXERCISE

STEP 1: **Take this survey to help you explore different angles of how you view your pregnant body.** Try to go with your gut, without censoring. You'll get the most accurate information that way.

Rate how much you agree with each statement:

1. My pregnancy feels like an alien invasion.
2. Sharing space with my baby is the most awesome thing that's ever happened to me.
3. I appreciate all that my body is doing for me and my baby.
4. I wish I could feel comfortable with the idea of sharing my body. It just creeps me out.
5. It's all about my baby. Sometimes I forget that there's a "me" in there at all.

STEP 2: **Write a brief reflection on the implications of the survey you just took.** For example, are you happy with your dominant view of your pregnant body? How does it match up with some of the research we looked at in the action component?

TIPS

Tip 1: Whatever you're feeling is just that – what you're feeling. Accept it and don't bash yourself, even if you are not all that thrilled about having a roommate – inside your body.

Celebrating the life I'm creating is abstract and weird.

I know that there is a life inside of me. I mean, if there wasn't I wouldn't be pregnant. And yet, celebrating the life inside me seems abstract and weird. It's definitely against my nature.

For:

1. It's not only weird, it's also a bad omen. How can you celebrate something that doesn't exist yet?
2. What's to celebrate? It's that little life inside me that's been me feel as though my body's been invaded by UFOs.
3. I'm just not one of these imaginative types. Different people can celebrate pregnancy in different ways. And that's okay!

Any other reason?

4. ____

Against:

1. Yeah, it's weird, but celebrating the life inside of me is something I could get behind in theory. Even if it feels foreign, I'm game to give it a try.
2. Seems like a great way to shift my mind from my body to my baby.
3. My baby is the realest thing to me right now. Imaginative or not, I plan to celebrate!

Why is it important for you to celebrate this new life?

4. ____

Imagination can help you love your pregnant body.

We all know those imaginative types. The ones who used to make dynasties out of carboard boxes as children and now, as adults, can still create universes in their minds. Well if you are one of those, then loving your pregnant body should be easy as 1-2-3.

For:

1. It's a cinch for me to close my eyes and visualize a crowd applauding for me as I strut my pregnant stuff down the catwalk.
2. I use my imagination to help me focus on what my body will look like after pregnancy, with my cute little baby and stroller in tow. It helps me love my pregnant body right now.
3. My imagination helps me stay out of my body, which is where I need to be right now!

Add your own idea:

4. ____

Against:

1. I might be imaginative, but that doesn't make me delusional. I know how to separate truth from reality.
2. Imaginative people have it worse – way worse – when it comes to loving their bodies. What they see when they look in the mirror has almost no basis in reality!
3. Imagination and positive body image are two separate skills. What does one have to do with the other?

Add your own idea:

4. ____

A pregnant woman should focus on anything *but* her baby.

Yeah, I get it. Pregnancy is about both mom and babe. But truth be told, I do better – and certainly feel better in my pregnant body – when I'm not thinking about my baby at all. Shouldn't women like me be making every effort to focus on anything *but* their babies?

For:

1. In order not to resent my baby for what it's doing to my body, it's best to separate my 'body' thoughts from my 'baby' thoughts as much as possible.
2. It's not my baby's fault I'm feeling large and uncomfortable. I don't want to bring him or her into the picture.
3. After the birth, I know it'll be all about baby. I need to focus on myself and on other things while I still can.

Why should you focus on things other than the baby?

4. ____

Against:

1. Focusing on my baby will bring down my levels of resentment. Ignoring my baby will create an environment where resentment will grow. It's like turning on the lights in a dark attic.
2. If I think about my growing body as a home, then I'll feel a lot more positive and purposeful about my body's changes.
3. Having a kid means learning to share. What begins with sharing my body will become sharing every facet of my life. I view pregnancy as my training period. Of course I need to think about the baby right now.

Add your own idea:

4. ____

The moment I realized this pregnancy wasn't just about me.

The experience of pregnancy is so connected to our physiology; it's not unusual to forget that we are now sharing our body with another human being! When did you realize that there was another person – a.k.a. baby – involved in this pregnancy? Take five minutes to write about that realization in your journal.

Direct message us YOUR story @Buddy_N_Soul on Instagram and be anonymously featured for a chance to **win a Buddy&Soul three month free membership**.

If I don't love my pregnant body yet, I'm never gonna

Much like being pregnant, loving your pregnant body is something that just is or isn't. If it's been a few months and you don't love your pregnant body yet, chances are nuttin's gonna make you start now. Here's why.

For:

1. My body is only getting bigger and more foreign. If I don't love my body like this, I'm not going to love it in a month's time. And certainly not by the end of my third trimester!
2. Loving my body, and my pregnant body, is an innate skill possessed by a lucky few.
3. If I've always struggled with positive image, why should I expect it to be any different (let alone any better) during pregnancy?
4. I've tried and haven't succeeded. It's time to give up.

Add your own:

5. ____

Against:

1. The closer I get to birth, the more I love my body because I can feel my baby so much more.
2. Loving my body is an acquired skill. If I haven't acquired it, I can continue to work on myself until I've got it in the bag.
3. It's not an all-or-nothing deal. Nothing in life is.

Add your own:

4. ____

What helps you feel attractive when you're pregnant?

We all have our own tricks to help us feel good in the skin we're in. What helps you feel attractive when you're pregnant?

1. Treating my body to something special, like a prenatal massage or even a manicure.
2. Standing in the mirror and pretending I'm on the cover of Vogue.
3. Exercising and eating well.
4. Sex with my partner.
5. Reminding myself that I have a baby inside me. What's more feminine than that?
6. Nada. I just don't feel attractive when I'm pregnant.

Add your own ideas to the list:

7. ____

8. ____

9. ____

STRATEGY 5: Appoint a voice of reason

When asked about what makes them happy, many millennials answer wealth and fame. But, according to a 70-year-long study out of Harvard, the *real* secret to long-term happiness is nothing material.

Spoiler alert: It all comes down to meaningful relationships.

And when you're pregnant, a meaningful relationship can be the one constant that help you reorient and find your way back to *you*.

Watch 'What makes a good life? Lessons from the longest study on happiness' presented by Robert Waldinger on YouTube.

As you watch this talk, think about the role that relationships play in your life, and whether there is someone whom you'd trust to help you navigate through the challenges of pregnancy.

The unexpected person who helped me love my pregnant body

Sometimes people in our lives help us see truths we've been denying. Were you surprised to learn that your pregnant body is worthy of your love? Think about the unexpected person who finally cracked your shell and got the message to sink in. Take a few moments with your journal to write about it.

Direct message us YOUR story @Buddy_N_Soul on Instagram and be anonymously featured for a chance to **win a Buddy&Soul three month free membership**.

DRIVING THE MESSAGE HOME

As any woman who's ever been pregnant will attest to, no matter how much you intend to remain cool, calm, and collected, at some point your emotions will get the better of your rational thought.

Some women are more affected than others, but nearly all will experience a ride or two on the emotional rollercoaster. And when this happens, it simply doesn't matter if you *know* that it's natural to gain weight, or break out, or sweat in places the Good Lord never intended a woman to sweat. What you *feel* is massively disgusting, and **you'll need a voice you trust to help you find north for times when you can't really trust yourself.**

Turn to someone you love and trust and officially appoint them your Voice of Reason. This can be a sister, a close friend, your partner, or anyone you trust to be there for you. Tell them (in advance if possible) that you are going to need them to help prevent and deal with body images issues as they arise.

Just don't expect them to read your mind. Not all well-meaning friends and partners will get it right without for-dummy instructions. Some people, for instance, don't understand intuitively that "Well, of course you're fat; you're pregnant!" is unhelpful.

(Plus: Check out our Relationship Saver During Pregnancy course )

And besides, different women like to hear different things. One woman will want to be reassured of how sexy she looks, and another reminded of the sacred function her body is serving.

To avoid well-intended but ill-received forms of encouragement, you may need to spell out precisely what you'll want to hear when things start heading downtown.

Of course, before you can share this information with your Voice of Reason, you'll first need to figure it out for yourself.

Reflecting on your personality and the types of statements that have and have not resonated in the past, you should be able to generate at least a few ideas of comments that would boost your body image and calm you down when you're in a body image rut.

You may wish to make a list that you can share with your Voice of Reason, with suggestions like, "It's only natural you feel uncomfortable, but to outside eyes you look amazing," or "You're beautiful. Do you think anyone will be looking at your ankles?"

Find what works for you and believe it when you hear it.

Finally, don't hesitate to ask your Voice of Reason to tell you these things in the course of your everyday life and not only when disaster strikes. Think of it as a hearty dose of preventive medicine.

Imagine you have a pregnancy fairy godmother who always knows just the right things to say. When you hit a body image slump, you simply wave your magic wand and she appears to make you feel beautiful again. What words does she say when you're feeling less-than-fabulous about your pregnant body?

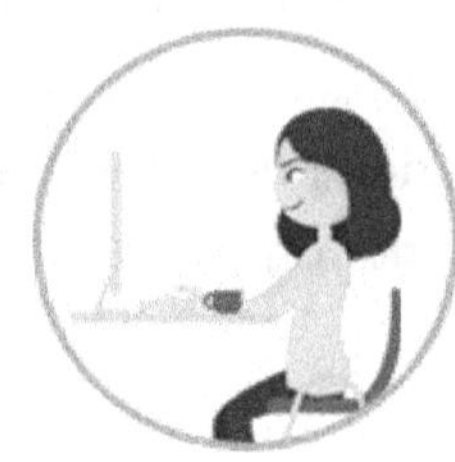

Write her brief script in your journal.

TIPS

Tip 1: Even if no one ever says these words aloud to you, it's helpful to know what you'd like to hear. In fact, why not read your fairy godmother's script to yourself on a daily basis?

Tip 2: Put a copy of this script in a prominent place so you remember to look it over frequently. You can even capture a screenshot and set it as the background for your phone.

9 Things (almost) every pregnant woman wants to hear

Although of course you are unique, and need reassurance that suits you, there are some phrases that almost no pregnant can resist. Find the ones you like and remind your loved ones to reassure you, frequently and passionately!

1. The changes in your body are amazing – they are helping you bring a child into the world.
2. Every single moment of your pregnancy is meaningful because you are creating life. You are never doing nothing.
3. You are *not* gaining weight for fun. You are pregnant!
4. No one's looking at your flaws – who can see past that maternal glow?
5. I hope you feel as good as you look. Because, dude, you look awesome.
6. Wow. Just wow.

Write some additional phrases that you want to hear:

7. ____

8. ____

9. ____

No one can help me love my pregnant body

I'm not loving my pregnant body, and I don't think any "Voice of Reason" can change that. I'm better off just waiting till the baby's out and I get my body back again before I try to start loving it. I mean, who are we kidding?

For:

1. Feeling good about yourself must come from within. Telling yourself that you love your pregnant body when you don't isn't going to change anything.
2. I grew up in a culture where thin was in, whether you were pregnant or not. It's difficult for me to embrace the weight gain that comes along with pregnancy, no matter how beautiful anyone else tells me I look.

Add your own ideas:

3. ____

Against:

1. The messages I hear in my environment really rub off on me. It would be amazing to hear positive messages about being pregnant and I think the right Voice of Reason really *could* make a difference.
2. The women I know who have already had babies have helped normalize the pregnancy experience for me. These girlfriends remind me to love and accept my body and that makes a difference in how I feel about myself.
3. When my partner tells me that my pregnant body is beautiful, and I can see that they really believe it, I start to believe it too.

Add your own ideas:

4. ____

How a voice of reason prevented body image mayhem

Various physical changes are an occupational hazard of pregnancy, from varicose veins to a swelling belly. How did someone you know help you find your way back home when your body image started to head downhill? Take some time to note this experience in your journal.

Direct message us YOUR story @Buddy_N_Soul on Instagram and be anonymously featured for a chance to **win a Buddy&Soul three month free membership**.

STRATEGY 6: Celebrate the things that stay the same

After years of struggling with body image,
Marla Mervis-Hartmann shares how she
managed to move away from the shame-based
"no pain, no gain" mentality and replace it with
what she calls "more pleasures, more
treasures."

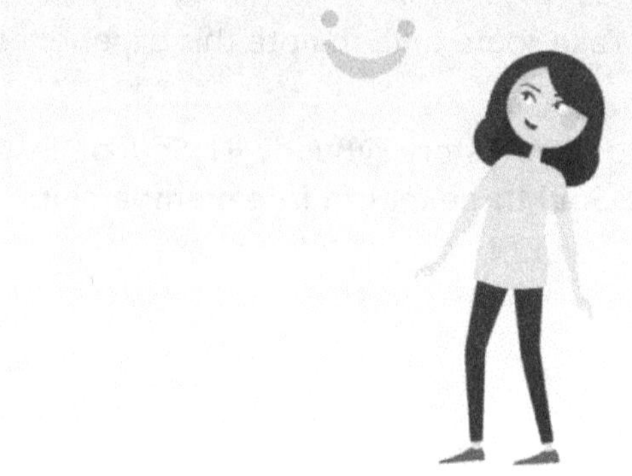

It is important to celebrate the things that you
find beautiful about yourself and your body.
The things that have remained unchanged through your pregnancy, or the new pleasant surprises that
have developed. And you can't do that unless you're willing to go there.

**Watch 'The Secret Ingredient to Feeling Good in your Body' presented by Marla Mervis-Hartmann at
TEDxSalinas on YouTube.**

As you watch, consider whether you're open to experiencing the treasures and pleasures that come
when you allow yourself to love your body – pregnant or not.

What's the secret ingredient to loving your pregnant body?

Having positive body image during pregnancy will make you feel better about yourself. What factors help you love your pregnant body?

1. Knowing that it's in my power to be happy with my body just the way it is.
2. Making the conscious choice to experience pleasure and enjoy my body sensations.
3. Moving my body in a loving way every day.
4. Letting food be a source of pleasure, not guilt or shame.
5. Telling myself positive messages about my body.

Add your secret ingredients:

6. ____

7. ____

8. ____

DRIVING THE MESSAGE HOME

By now, you've likely been told that everything about your body will change. Not just your belly, but your thighs, hips, bust, arms, ankles...everything.

But remember that in pregnancy, only *almost* everything changes; many things do actually stay the same. If you can learn to focus on these things, it'll make it easier to view your pregnant body in a more positive light and to get through the times when nothing else feels pretty.

You might want to focus, say, on your hazel eyes, or on your beautiful eyelashes; you might paint your nails a fun color that makes you happy every time you catch a glimpse of your hands. If you're one of lucky ones whose shoe size hasn't changed during pregnancy, consider investing in a pretty-yet-comfortable pair of pregnancy-friendly flats that will also serve you well once the baby is born.

Yes, these seemingly insignificant gestures can improve how you feel about your pregnant body, shallow though they may appear.

Because, **while you can't control all of your body's big changes, you *can* hold onto parts of you that still make you feel beautiful.** And you should – because chances are, you've got a lot more going for you than you realize.

EXERCISE

Pick one part of you that will not be affected by pregnancy, **take a quick pic to remind yourself of one of your favorite, unchanging features**. Come back to this image any time you feel like your body image is spiraling out of control. Share your experience with loving your pregnant body and then share your story with the Buddy and Soul community! Tag us on Instagram and Twitter @Buddy_N_Soul, using the #BuddynSoulExpecting. By sharing with us on social media, not only can you help others with their personal journeys, you can read about those facing similar challenges.

TIPS

Tip 1: Feel free to come back to this exercise and keep adding more and more pics of all your wonderful features – both those that are changing with your pregnancy and those that are not. This can become like a photo journal and a powerful way to boost your pregnant ego.

11 Fun ways to feel great about your pregnant body

It won't last forever, so find some fun ways to enjoy your pregnant body and revel in the experience! Here are a few ideas for starters.

1. Make a belly cast and decorate it as a keepsake of your pregnancy.
2. Hang out with a pregnant friend and share pregnancy stories.
3. Keep a photo log of your growing belly on a regular basis, whether daily, weekly or monthly, and you'll have an unforgettable record of your baby's growth before birth.
4. Watch a fun pregnancy movie. Or two. Or ten.
5. Pamper yourself with a sensory experience that you love. Perhaps a bubble bath, scented candles, or a massage.
6. Go out and buy something new, maternity style.
7. Join a pregnancy exercise or yoga group.
8. Take pregnancy portraits with your partner.

Do you have any other suggestions?

9. ____

10. ____

11. ____

(Plus: Check out our Relationship Saver During Pregnancy course for more awesome relationship-building ideas.)

What makes you feel beautiful during pregnancy

Some of us feel like we're glowing, and others yearn for our pre-pregnancy shape. Regardless, we all want to feel beautiful, and so we should! What makes you feel beautiful during pregnancy?

1. Flattering maternity clothes.
2. Receiving positive feedback from my partner, friends, and acquaintances.
3. Feeling grateful that I'm pregnant.
4. A prenatal boudoir photo shoot!
5. Wearing my favorite jewelry.

Add your own ideas:

6. ____

7. ____

8. ____

What feeling beautiful during pregnancy looks like for me

Most of us want to feel beautiful, whether we're pregnant or not! When you consider all the changes that are happening inside and outside of your body, how have you adjusted your view of beauty this pregnancy? Write down some of your adjustments in your journal.

STRATEGY 7: Show your pregnant body you care

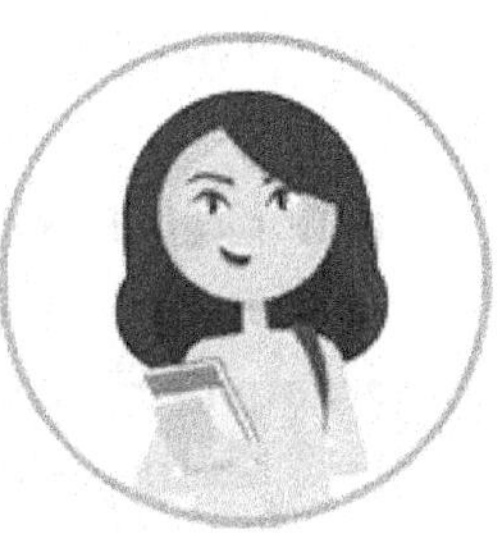

Tracey Spicer, a radio and television journalist, talks about the time and effort that women invest in their daily grooming routines. She points out some surprising statistics about grooming and productivity and argues that all that wasted time would be much better spent achieving and doing things we actually care about!

What does your beauty regimen look like, normally and now that you're pregnant? Are you over-grooming, aka obsessing, or are you putting reasonable efforts into feeling good about yourself and boosting your self-esteem?

Watch 'The Lady Stripped Bare' presented by Tracey Spicer from TEDxSouthBankWomen on YouTube.

Spicer certainly leaves us with some fascinating food for thought!

STRATEGY 7: Show your pregnant body you care

Should I trim my beauty regimen during pregnancy?

In her TED Talk *The Lady Stripped Bare*, Australian journalist and news personality Tracey Spicer encourages women to use their time more efficiently by dropping various parts of their morning grooming rituals. Some people may find that extremely hard to do, especially during pregnancy! But it may just be worth the effort.

For:

1. I'm already feeling insecure. How would *dropping* my grooming help?
2. I don't want to fall short of societal expectations, no matter how objectively ridiculous they are.
3. My exercise, makeup, and grooming routines keep me feeling in control when there's so much during pregnancy that makes me feel *out* of control.

How would keeping your beauty regimen help you during pregnancy?

4. ____

Against:

1. I feel amazing when I am more natural. And I love seeing other women being more natural as well. It lets me feel *less* shame, because I'm not using makeup as a mask.
   (For more on the masks we hide behind, check out our Cultivating Authenticity course)
2. As women, we put far too much pressure on ourselves. This isn't even about feminism – it's about allowing ourselves to be more comfortable in the skin we're in.
3. I would trim or even drop my beauty regimen if it meant that I'd have more time for important things! Especially with the baby coming, I'll need as much extra time as possible.

How would trimming your beauty regimen help you during pregnancy?

4. ____

DRIVING THE MESSAGE HOME

Whether you're young or a bit older, female or male, pregnant or not, appearance does matter; you always want to put your best foot forward. But your body is not just something to *look* at – it's your vehicle for moving around in and interacting with the world.

It's your most dependable friend. It does so much for you and deserves to feel the love! And yet, many times, if you're like me at least, you might not treat your body with the respect and compassion it deserves for all its hard work.

Showing your body you care means taking care of it even when you don't feel like it. It means doing those grown-up things that you know are important for your body, and especially important during pregnancy, like eating well, exercising, flossing, drinking plenty of water, staying on top of any meds or supplements you've been prescribed, and of course, getting enough sleep. Even moisturizing your skin falls under the category of pregnancy self-care.

(Plus: Check out our Sticking to Your Pregnancy Plan course 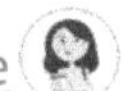)

While all forms of self-care will contribute to a healthy pregnancy, let's talk a little more about the importance of exercising, with your physician's okay of course.

Our bodies are made to move, even and maybe especially during pregnancy. And not only that, prenatal exercise is actually positively correlated with body image.

A study done by researchers at the University of Melbourne found that women who exercised during pregnancy usually had more positive feelings towards their body and had a greater sense of psychological wellbeing.

Along similar lines, a Canadian study found that exercise played an important role in pregnant women's wellbeing, mitigating fatigue, anxiety, and depression.

In fact, study after study replicates this finding in one form or another: **exercise is an important part of a healthy mom-to-be, a healthy baby, and a healthy pregnancy.** With the help of your doctor, you can plan a safe and enjoyable exercise routine for your pregnancy.

There are infinite ways to show your pregnant body you care. This session is about finding what works best for you.

EXERCISE

Make a list of things that you can do for your pregnant body. This can be buying a new pair of comfortable walking shoes, using nourishing lotions for your skin, taking a healing bubble bath, drinking healthy smoothies, or switching to eye make-up for sensitive eyes. Anything that is good for your pregnant body will be good for you. Make sure to include a form of exercise that you can do to make your body feel great, pending doctoral approval.

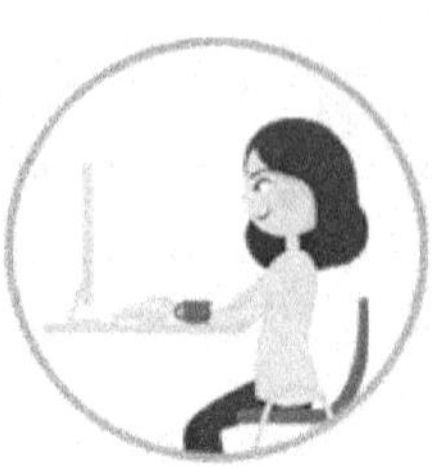

TIPS

Tip 1: Use the list to get you going. Yes, today – why not? Your body deserves it!

Tip 2: You can research some great pregnancy self-care product suggestions. Check them out!

10 Ways to show your pregnant body you care

Taking care of your body sends the message that you accept it and will not subject it to unrealistic societal expectations. Not sure how to start? Here are a few ideas to inspire you.

1. Drinking water and healthy, energizing juices or smoothies.
2. Following a daily prenatal exercise routine (at the approval of your doctor or midwife, of course).
3. Getting yourself comfortable shoes, some good new bras, and maternity clothing that fits you well.
4. Switching to sensitive, chemical-free cosmetic and skin-care products.
5. Finding healthier alternatives for your meals or snacks.
6. Taking naps!
7. Engaging in active, daily relaxation practices (breathing, outdoor walking, yoga, mindfulness, etc.).

Any other ideas?

8. ____

9. ____

10. ____

Prenatal exercise is for Type A mamas.

We all know those Type A mamas and mamas-to-be. The ones who you just know will be nursing in a perfectly ironed button-down shirt from day one. Well, those are the type that'll succeed at prenatal exercise. For the rest of us normal folks, it's nothing more than a pipe dream.

For:

1. The whole idea of committing to anything besides my bed gives me the heebie-jeebies.
2. Who can think about exercise between the all-day "morning" sickness and juggling the responsibilities of regular life, plus a million prenatal appointments? Clearly, only a Type A mom-to-be. Not I.
3. You need to know how to make a decision and stick with it in order to succeed at prenatal exercise. Only uber-conscientious folks can do that. Again, not I.

Add your own idea:

4. ____

Against:

1. The studies don't discriminate based on personality: prenatal exercise is beneficial for *all* women – not just for Type A women.
2. Exercise and other health behaviors during pregnancy are my choice to make. I may have to work harder than some other women to make exercise happen, but it's still a choice that's available to me.

Add your own idea:

3. ____

What happened when I started showing my pregnant body the love

Many pregnancies are accompanied by challenging physiological side effects. We know that properly caring for our bodies can help us feel much better. Did you notice a difference in the way you felt after you started treating your body with love and respect? Use your journal to write down some of the ways you cared for your body and how you felt afterwards.

Direct message us YOUR story @Buddy_N_Soul on Instagram and be anonymously featured for a chance to **win a Buddy&Soul three month free membership**.

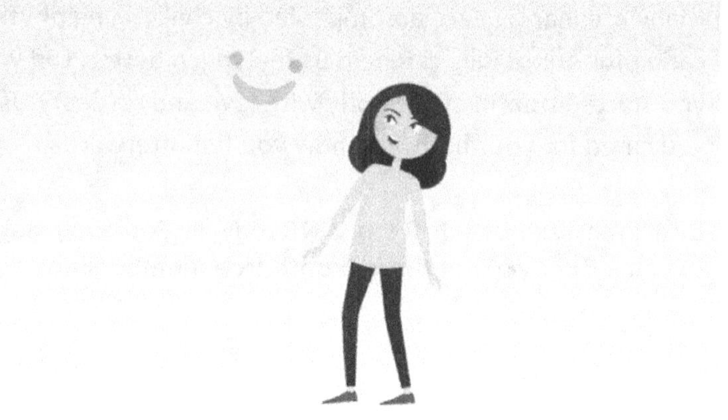

Watch 'Living Without Shame: How We Can Empower Ourselves' presented by Whitney Thore from TEDxGreensboro on YouTube.

In the TED Talk presented by Whitney Way Thore, the star of TLC's My Big Fat Fabulous Life, she tells us about her journey through shame, eating disorders, PCOS, and weight gain; and then how she turned her life around, not by losing weight but by accepting herself, living authentically, and building confidence, no matter what others said about her.

We can learn a valuable lesson from this: what others say doesn't define us. It our beliefs, reactions, and choices that determine our reality.

(Plus: Check out our Cultivating Authenticity course 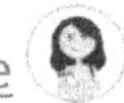)

10 Tips for living without body shame during pregnancy

Comments about our bodies, whether said innocently or intentionally, can sting. This is especially true during pregnancy when many women are extra vulnerable about their body's changes. Here are some tips to get you started on living shame-free when it comes to your pregnant body.

1. The more you praise yourself, the more you will believe that you are worthy of praise. Praise your beautiful baby belly, your pregnancy glow, and even the parts of your body that you can't see but are doing such a great job of nurturing your baby.
2. When you live your own life (including your private thoughts) without shame, then the opinions of others have no effect.
3. Acknowledge shame you feel around your pregnant body. Sounds counterintuitive, but shame grows when we ignore it and dissipates when we let it know we've heard it out.
4. Talk back to your inner critic. If there are others putting you down, don't let your inner critic get in on the action. You may not be able to yell "back off!" to a boss or friend who makes a stinging remark about your changing body, but you *can* talk back to your own inner critic.
5. Live your life, even if you feel self-conscious. Don't let others' hurtful comments about your looks stop you from enjoying your life. *Everyone* is entitled to live their lives!
6. Weed out bad friends. A one-off thoughtless comment about your pregnant body can be excused, but if there is someone in your life who makes you feel bad regularly and on purpose, you may want to take a look at the relationship.
7. Adopt a positive mantra that makes you feel good about your body during pregnancy and beyond (e.g., I am beautiful, I am confident, I am strong and don't care what others say).

Add your own:

8. ____

9. ____

10. ____

DRIVING THE MESSAGE HOME

Even those of us who do not regularly engage in swordplay often find ourselves needing to suddenly defend ourselves against jabbing comments during pregnancy.

A friend might say, "OMG, you're huge! It's crazy, you're normally so thin but now you're like…like…" and while she casts about for the perfect metaphor to express just how *vast* you've gotten, you're expected to stand there and smile politely, and perhaps even supply the image she was looking for. "A python digesting a wildebeest?" "Exactly!" she'll cry happily, and then continue to take polite interest in your health.

The field of Dialectical Behavior Therapy, or DBT, teaches that while you can't control what people say, you *can* control how you react.

Let's suppose you're a preschool teacher and one of your charming little young'uns innocently asks why you were skinny before the holidays and now you're so big (true story).

Some will take this innocent-but-offensive comment to heart and spiral right into guilt and shame mode – as if we were talking about having eaten too much ice cream and not about a baby gestating in there!

Others will laugh it off and let it roll like water off a duck's back.

The difference, according to DBT, is in the interpretation. *You* choose whether you hear "Hey Teach, what in the world did you do to turn into a mammoth over the past two weeks!?" Or, "I'm five years old, curious about the world, and haven't quite learned the fine art of social subtlety just yet."

By arming yourself in advance with some possible reinterpretations of stinging remarks about your pregnant body, you won't be frozen in shock when someone says something you'd rather they hadn't.

Good options might be, "They've got no idea what a pregnancy entails," or "If they knew how offensive I'd find that, they'd never say it," or, "They're entitled to their opinions, and I'm entitled to ignore them."

This is true for comments made innocently with no malicious intent. When it comes to spiteful, intentionally insulting comments, it's harder to let the sting slide. Nonetheless, it helps to keep in mind that people's comments about your body often stem from their own insecurities, not objective truths about how you look (see *Does This Pregnancy Make Me Look Fat?* p. 191 for more). In those cases, all you can do is remind yourself that this is about them, not about you, and move on.

So, the next time you're met with a cringe-worthy remark that has the potential to strike a serious blow to your body image, remember to check your interpretations before you yell *en garde* and save yourself a lot of aggravation.

EXERCISE

Pick one cringe-worthy comment you've heard about a pregnant woman's looks (whether yours, someone else's, or even a book, movie, or TV character's). And if no one commented, think of something you dread hearing. Note it in your journal.

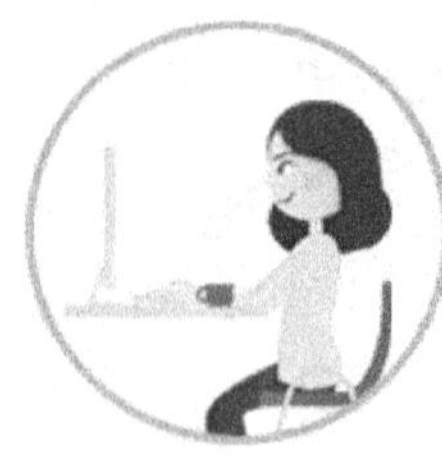

Below it, **write out at least one more generous alternative interpretation you can ascribe to this biting remark.** So, instead of 'everyone thinks I'm huge!' why not go with the equally valid 'people make silly and unfounded statements sometimes'?

TIPS

Tip 1: If you liked this exercise in reinterpretation, be sure to check out our Everyday Reframing course. 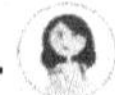

Tip 2: This shouldn't take you more than a few minutes and will likely be invaluable next time someone says something you can't believe you actually just heard (which will hopefully be never)!

10 Great reframes for rude comments about your pregnant body

Once you hit a certain point in your pregnancy, comments like 'you look huge,' or 'are you having twins?' can become commonplace. Here are some great ways to reframe those comments and reclaim positive feelings about your pregnant body.

(For more on reframing, check out our course on it!)

1. The giver of the dumb comment did not mean anything negative. They simply don't know how to pay a compliment.
2. If they're making such a dumb comment, they must think I have really high self-esteem because I look so friggin' gorgeous.
3. 'Sticks and stones may break my bones but words will never hurt me.'
4. All that matters is how I think and feel about myself.
5. What? Can't hear ya. Did you say I look fiiiiine?
6. *I* know that I am doing everything that I can in my pregnancy. Stupid comments are not a reflection of reality.
7. Yes, I'm getting bigger, which just means there's more of my awesomeness in this universe.

Add your own ideas to the list:

8. ____

9. ____

10. ____

What helps you ignore stinging remarks about your pregnant body?

Some days it may be easier and other days harder, but you *can* brush off hurtful jabs about your pregnant body. Here are some things that may help you not take them to heart.

1. Knowing there's someone out there who disagrees.
2. Knowing that *I* disagree.
3. Knowing it was meant as a harmless joke, even if it hurt me.
4. Reminding myself of all the hurtful comments I've made to others.
5. Remembering that everyone is allowed to have human moments and to make mistakes.
6. Nothing. This is really hard for me to do.

Anything else?

7. ____

8. ____

9. ____

The hands-down dumbest comment I got during my pregnancy

When you are the recipient of one of these comments, jaw hits the table and you're appalled that people can say such dumb things. Well… it happens. Here's your chance to brainstorm in your journal about some of the absolute dumbest pregnancy comments that you or someone you know received.

STRATEGY 9: Enjoy the present of the present

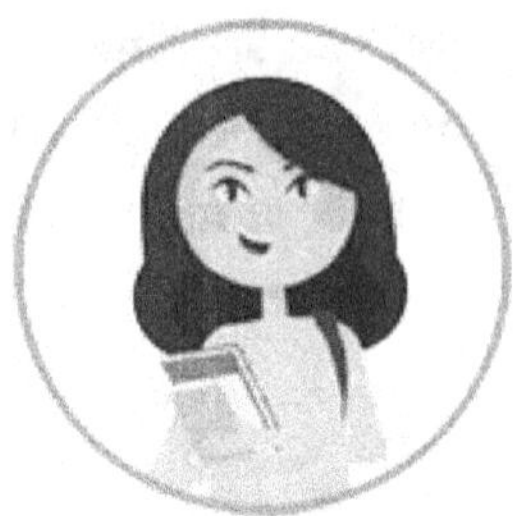

In an act of courage, even social subversion, Kelli Jean Drinkwater challenges our perceptions of where bigger bodies are "allowed." She invites us to rethink how we engage with bigger bodies – whether our own or others' – and encourages us to drop the apologetics around being big.

Her work is a response to the 'fatphobia' of our culture, where we equate fat with bad and thin with good.

Watch 'Enough with the Fear of Fat' presented by Kelli Jean Drinkwater on YouTube.

As you listen to Drinkwater, apply her words to your own pregnancy and fears. Ask yourself if you are allowing the fear of being big to harm you and your baby during your pregnancy.

Does your fear of weight gain affect your pregnancy?

Many women are concerned about how much weight they will gain and how that will affect them and their babies. To what extent are you concerned about the flashing number on your scale?

1. I know that healthy weight gain is a natural part of pregnancy.
2. I am worried that I will never get my pre-baby body back.
3. I dread getting stretch marks as my belly swells.
4. I consider my food options carefully for the health of my baby.
5. I'm concerned that I'm not gaining enough weight.

Anything else?

6. ____

7. ____

8. ____

DRIVING THE MESSAGE HOME

A pregnancy lasts nine months. Maybe a tad into the tenth. But then it ends. And it doesn't come back. So, why do so many of us moms-to-be have a hard time enjoying the ride?

The science in this area suggests that many of us are just too busy worrying about how we'll get our bodies back after the baby is born! Sounds silly? Perhaps, but it's true.

One study found that during pregnancy, women believe their bodies to be "transgressing the socially constructed ideal" of what they *should* look like. It's as if they feel they're letting society down by taking up more space than they're supposed to, just by gaining the basic weight needed for a healthy mom and healthy baby.

The anxiety doesn't stop after delivery. Oh no. It can continue well into the post-partum period when, according to psychotherapist Susie Orbach and body image expert Holli Rubin, a new mom is expected to "present herself physically as though nothing as momentously life-changing or body-changing as having a baby has occurred" (p.5). And that is hardly short of absurd!

If you are anything like the women in these studies, it's time to switch gears. Because, **when you're busy dreading the impacts pregnancy will have on your future figure, you don't have much time or energy left to enjoy the benefits of the present.**

Alternatively, making an effort to view your pregnancy as a fun and special time will take a major load off and will positively impact your body image too.

A few ideas of ways to enjoy the special perks of your pregnancy are:

- Go on dates with your partner, even on a romantic getaway
- Take guilt-free naps and go to bed as early as you please
- Sign up for an awesome prenatal yoga or fitness class
- Enjoy watching your personal TV as your baby kicks and your belly moves
- Get a pregnancy massage
- Accept offers of help from friends, family, colleagues, and even strangers

In short, do whatever you can to help spin your entire pregnancy experience in a more positive light. While no one's going to give you a hard-and-fast guarantee of what your body will look like in a year's time – and yes, you may still be lugging around some extra pounds – the good news is that all anyone expects you to do right now is make responsible, healthy choices. Nothing more, and certainly nothing extreme.

So, why not stop and smell the roses? Enjoy the present of the present without lugging around the extra weight (so to speak) of what your future will hold.

(Plus: Check out our Mindfulness for Beginners course 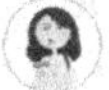)

The more positively you view your pregnancy right now, the more at peace you'll feel with your present and future body.

EXERCISE

What's your favorite perk of being pregnant? Maybe it's the fact that your belly doubles as a nightstand, or the opportunity you now have to wear those A-line dresses that usually don't flatter your body type. Maybe it's the proverbial pregnancy "glow" you're actually seeing in your own face! Whatever it is, **use your journal to write about it.** Then share your story with the Buddy and Soul community! Take a picture and tag us on Instagram and Twitter @Buddy_N_Soul, using the #BuddynSoulExpecting. By sharing with us on social media, not only can you help others with their personal journeys, you can read about those facing similar challenges.

TIPS

Tip 1: Come back to this page in your journal whenever you feel like there's nothing at all that could possibly be good about being pregnant. Not that any pregnant woman ever feels that way...

Tip 2: For more on enjoying your pregnancy as an opportunity to bond with your partner, check out our Relationship Saver During Pregnancy course.

11 Things you'll miss about being pregnant

Chances are that pregnancy has invited many new experiences into your life, some of which you'll really miss! Here are a few examples. Can you think of more?

1. Those special moments of bonding time with your partner, cuddling, and dreaming about the baby-to-be.
2. Having pregnancy as an excuse to miss all the events you didn't want to go to anyway.
3. Since being tired is your new reality, you can take guilt-free naps, every day. Even twice a day.
4. You can eat whatever you like and blame it on the "cravings."
5. Having a great conversation starter, wherever you go!
6. Perfect strangers help you carry your groceries and give you their seats on the subway.
7. That feeling of connection when you feel the baby moving.
8. Lowered expectations for almost everything.

What else will you miss?

9. ____

10. ____

11. ____

What are your favorite pregnancy perks?

Being pregnant is a stage that won't last forever, as we all know, so let's live it up! What do you love most about being pregnant?

1. Positive attention from absolute strangers.
2. Loving my growing belly.
3. Bonding with my partner.
4. Big shirts and loose clothing.
5. You can blame everything on hormones.

List other perks you enjoy:

6. ____

7. ____

8. ____

When I focused on enjoying my pregnancy, better body image followed

We all want to be present in our lives, which, during pregnancy, means taking the time to slow down and enjoy the ride. Write about it in your journal. How did your body image improve when you started enjoying your pregnancy?

Direct message us YOUR story @Buddy_N_Soul on Instagram and be anonymously featured for a chance to **win a Buddy&Soul three month free membership**.

STRATEGY 10: Thank your body for carrying you through pregnancy

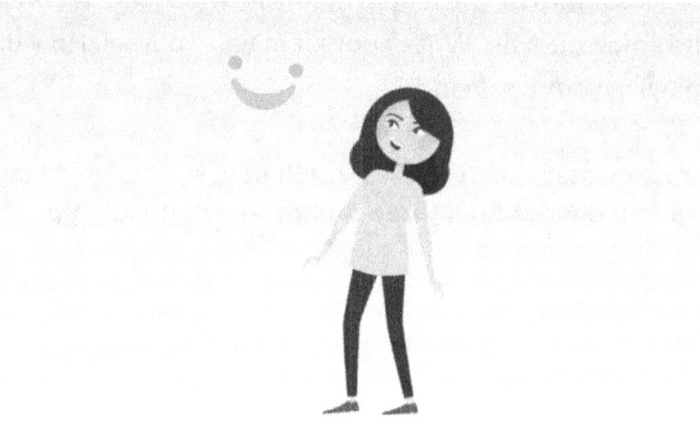

Image-maker Alexander Tsiaras shares a powerful medical digital visualization, showing human development from conception to birth and beyond. His powerful images will truly take your breath away and help you experience, in a new way, how your body is creating life right now.

By taking a moment to pause and appreciate your life-giving abilities, you can cultivate gratitude towards your pregnant body: the body that's doing so much for you and your baby right now!

Watch 'Conception to birth – visualized' presented by Alexandra Tsiaras on www.ted.com.

12 Facts about pregnancy that will take your breath away

Pregnancy can truly take your breath away, if you stop to think about it. Here are a few facts that attest to the awesomeness of this very special time.

1. Your total cardiac output and blood volume increases by 30 – 50% during pregnancy.
2. By the end of your pregnancy, the uterus will have expanded to nearly 500 times its original size!
3. Did you know that four women give birth each second? There. Four women just gave birth.
4. From 18 weeks, your baby can hear and begins to respond to sensory input.
5. Although extremely rare, it is possible to get pregnant while pregnant! It's called superfetation.
6. Your baby's fingerprints are fully formed by 12 weeks in utero.
7. Baby girls develop all their reproductive eggs in utero. Boys wait until puberty to develop sperm.
8. Your feet can grow an entire shoe size during pregnancy, due to extra weight and fluid retention.
9. A heightened sense of smell can be a sign that you are pregnant – often before your pregnancy test will turn up positive!

What are some of the most fascinating facts that you have heard?

10. ____

11. ____

12. ____

DRIVING THE MESSAGE HOME

Regardless of whether this pregnancy was planned, spontaneous, or even desired, there is no denying the miracle you're currently part of. Pregnancy and birth are miraculous – each individual bit is so phenomenal if you stop to think about it. From conception all the way to the end, every step is something to marvel at and to be grateful for. So, let's end the book with a note of gratitude. Literally.

According to a study by the School of Applied Psychology at the University College of Cork, Ireland, gratitude during pregnancy is "correlated with positive affect, life satisfaction and pregnancy uplifts" (p. 665). In other words, **when you're pregnant, expressing gratitude towards your body and yourself has a positive impact on your mood and wellbeing.**

Sure, talking to your body in order to express gratitude sounds a bit cray cray, but bear with us.

And keep in mind that this doesn't have to mean a full-on heart-to-heart. Simple statements of gratitude will do.

For instance, things like, 'Thank you for knowing what to do without anyone telling you,' 'Thank you for housing this life inside of me,' and 'Thank you for giving me an excuse to finally put on some weight without feeling guilty.'

Whatever feels authentic to you, no matter how small or seemingly insignificant, focus there.

If you can overcome your initial bashfulness, you'll likely find this expression of gratitude a very powerful exercise.

EXERCISE

Write a letter of thanks in your journal to your body. Detail all the amazing things it has done, both for you and for your baby.

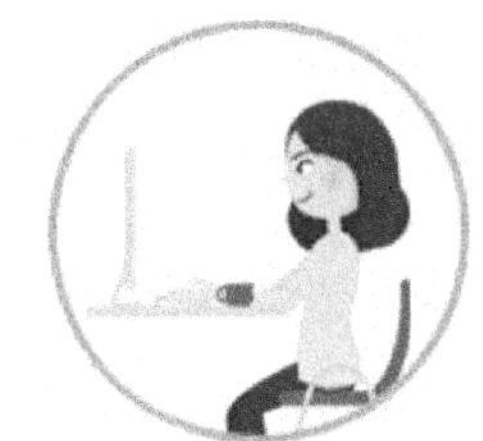

Direct message us YOUR letter @Buddy_N_Soul on Instagram and be anonymously featured for a chance to **win a Buddy&Soul three month free membership**.

TIPS

Tip 1: Is writing really not your thing? How about just writing "thanks" on your belly and snapping a selfie instead? Share your picture with the Buddy and Soul community! Tag us on Instagram and Twitter @Buddy_N_Soul, using the #BuddynSoulExpecting. By sharing with us on social media, not only can you help others with their personal journeys, you can read about those facing similar challenges.

Tip 2: Focusing on your baby may help you cultivate more gratitude than if you focus exclusively on your body.

Tip 3: This is your chance to really explore the many reasons you have to be grateful to your pregnant body. Think about everything it's done for you this pregnancy from digesting your food, to getting those supersized boobs you've always dreamed of, to creating a life!

Tip 4: We hope you enjoyed this book. Continue to check back in your journal periodically. The work you did throughout this book will serve as a sort of pregnancy scrapbook for you to look back on and smile.

8 Reasons to thank your body for your pregnancy

If you find yourself falling victim to negative thoughts about your pregnant body, try turning on the gratitude switch and see what a difference it makes. Here are some reasons to thank your body this pregnancy.

1. You have a human being growing inside of you. Enough said.
2. You are part of an eternal chain of life, including women who have done this before you and women who will do this after you.
3. You are able to become pregnant and to sustain a pregnancy. Sadly, many women in the world do not share your good fortune.
4. You can feel your baby kicking inside of you. And if you can't yet, you will soon!
5. Your body knows just what to do. With no intervention from you, your body duplicates your baby's cells at lightning speed, grows a placenta and an amniotic sac, and expands your uterus to fit your growing baby. If that doesn't deserve a shout-out, I don't know what does!

What are some other reasons to be thankful for your pregnancy?

6. ____

7. ____

8. ____

What inspires you to be grateful for your pregnancy

Cultivating gratitude for your pregnancy can help you improve your body image and your overall wellbeing. It's a win-win. So, what inspires *you* to feel thankful for your pregnancy?

1. My baby kicking inside of me.
2. Thinking about what the future will look like.
3. My ultrasound images.
4. Reminding myself that I'm part of a miracle.
5. Thinking about my desire to be a mom.
6. Inspired and grateful? No way!

What else inspires you?

7. ____

8. ____

9. ____

What happened when I chose to be grateful for my pregnant body

Research in positive psychology tells us that being grateful is good for you on so many levels. Was there a time when you felt deep gratitude for your pregnant body? Use your journal to write about it, and what positive effects followed.

Direct message us YOUR story @Buddy_N_Soul on Instagram and be anonymously featured for a chance to **win a Buddy&Soul three month free membership**.

10 Statements you'll hear from women who love their pregnant bodies

Lady, you were born for this. When you're floating through your pregnancy in an endorphin-induced blissful state, here are some things that you might say.

1. I love that my body is doing what it's made to do. I've never felt so empowered as a woman!
2. How awesome do these new curves look?
3. Isn't it great that I'm SUPPOSED to have a stomach that pokes out?
4. My baby is loving it in there. Guess I'm just a super comfortable person to hang out in.
5. Gosh, pregnancy really suits me. I should just stay pregnant and skip the postpartum stage!
6. I look totally hot. My partner is so freaking lucky.
7. My baby kicking me reminds me that I have a little buddy with me at all times. That is pretty awesome.

What other phrases might you hear from these empowered women?

8. ____

9. ____

10. ____

WHERE DO WE GO FROM HERE?

You've finished the Loving Your Pregnant Body book, but you haven't finished the journey. It doesn't end, it just gets better. Revisit this book, carry its ideas with you. Check out BuddynSoul.com and the rest of our books for all we have to offer. Spread the word. And change your life for good.

Sticking to Your Pregnancy Plan

You're having a baby (yay!) and you want everything to go smoothly. Following your doctor's orders concerning medication, vitamins, lifestyle changes, and diet is an important part of the plan…but that sure as heck ain't to say it's easy.

This book offers you a fresh new look at sticking to your medical provider's prenatal "rules." We'll explore the cognitive, emotional, and behavioral elements that can help you improve your health outcomes, and of course, your baby's.

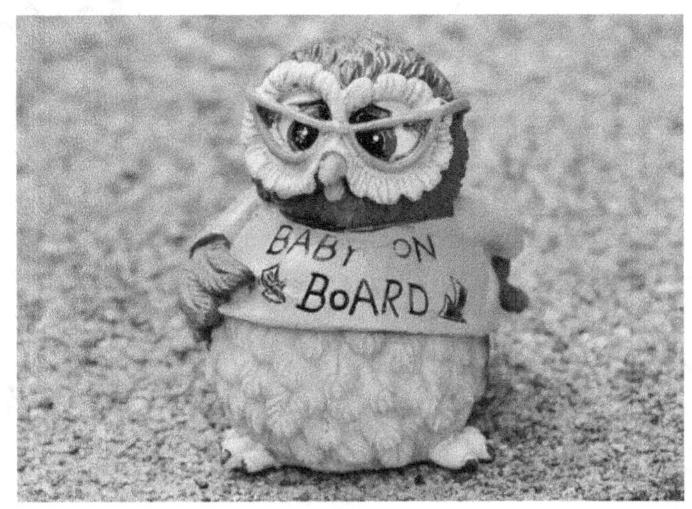

Goals you can achieve by reading 'Sticking to Your Pregnancy Plan':

1. Assume responsibility for sticking to your pregnancy health regimen.
2. Delve deeply into what may be holding you back from properly adhering to a healthy pregnant lifestyle.
3. Implement practical, research-based tools to help improve your adherence to your pregnancy plan.

Relationship Saver During Pregnancy

Pregnancy can put a strain on even the best relationships. That's why it's so important to preemptively support your relationship now, so your new family can be built on rock-solid foundations. Keeping in mind your needs, your partner's needs, and the needs of your relationship, this course will give you the know-how to strengthen your connection during pregnancy and beyond.

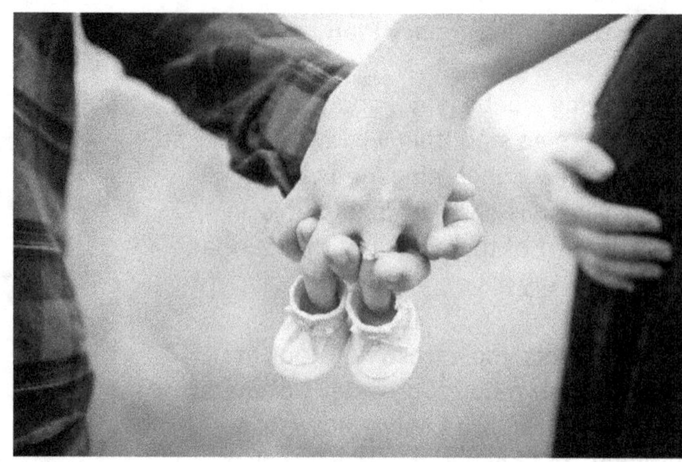

Goals you can achieve by reading 'Relationship Saver During Pregnancy':

1. Identify your needs – both as two individuals and as a pair – as you navigate this pregnancy.
2. Strengthen your communication and build your connection with your partner.
3. Take responsibility for improving your relationship during pregnancy and beyond.

Acing The Fourth Trimester
It is a universally acknowledged truth that much like a Jane Austen novel ends with a wedding, once you give birth and go home with a baby you end up at home with a new baby.

And experience pure bliss.

Now, back to reality. Considering that you're still hormonal and bleeding, possibly recovering from surgery or stitching, and your baby basically is a fetus with a vocal range that

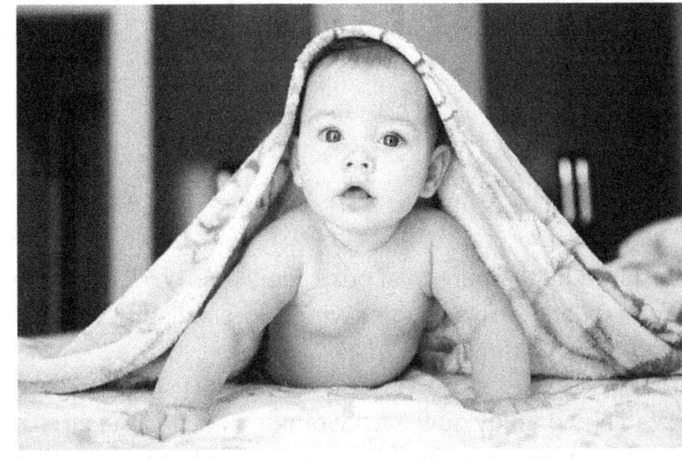

suddenly carries, it's not surprising that the first three months after birth are referred to as the "fourth trimester." Unfortunately, the books, websites, and apps seem to stop after three; those that *do* discuss the first year, focus almost solely on the newborn. Once the baby's out you're no longer a part of the pregnancy community, but you're not quite a part of the parenting fold, either. And you're certainly not back to your old self – with sleep, habits, stress, anything and everything that a tiny creature can and will throw off (but aren't they cute?).

That's where we come in. Join us to learn how to juggle this time of emotional ups and downs, of changing relationships, habits, and priorities. No matter how your baby came into the world, you're indisputably handling a lot more than you used to. We'll provide you with the tools you need to ace the fourth trimester, making your postnatal adjustment smoother, easier, and more enjoyable.

Goals you can achieve by reading 'Acing the Fourth Trimester:

1. Process your birth experience, whether it was positive, negative, or somewhere in the middle,
2. Learn strategies to help ease the difficult parts of your fourth trimester,
3. Help you create a post-birth roadmap to get you back to you.

WANT TO LEARN MORE? CHECK THESE OUT!

MOVIES

What to Expect When You're Expecting (2012)

Inspired by the perennial bestseller, *What to Expect When You're Expecting* is a hilarious and heartfelt comedy about five couples whose intertwined lives are turned upside down by the challenges of impending parenthood.

Watch and enjoy how each woman manages the gifts and challenges of pregnancy and motherhood, including the struggle of feeling good in her pregnant body.

40 Weeks (2014)

40 Weeks is the first unscripted documentary film to offer an intimate window into the week-by-week journey of pregnant women across the country.

40 Weeks explores the emotional and physical changes of pregnancy, the hopes and fears, and the confusing and often difficult choices that can be presented during this time.

MORE VIDEOS

Cameron Russell: Looks aren't everything. Believe me, I'm a model

Cameron Russell admits she won "a genetic lottery:" she's tall, pretty and an underwear model. But don't judge her by her looks. In this fearless talk, she takes a wry look at the industry that had her looking highly seductive at barely 16 years old.

An eye-opening talk for pregnant women who are constantly bombarded with problematic media images of what their pregnant bodies *should* look like.

Plus-size? More Like My Size | Ashley Graham | TEDxBerkleeValencia

Internationally-known body activist, model, and entrepreneur Ashley Graham describes her journey into fashion industry stardom. She doesn't leave out any of the gritty details as she describes the challenging and rewarding progression toward becoming her own role model. Inspiring body confidence in the next generation, Ashley expresses the need for the universal embrace of body diversity as beauty paradigms continue to shift.

An empowering talk for pregnant women who just want to be given the permission to embrace their growing and changing bodies!

BOOKS

The Bodies of Mothers: A Beautiful Body Project, by Jade Beall

You and your pregnant body are beautiful; now's the time to embrace what real, un-airbrushed, authentic women look like!

Based on real photographs of real people, enjoy this first book in a series that promotes the message of celebrating the irreplaceable beauty of women and the body positive movement happening all over the world.

Does This Pregnancy Make Me Look Fat?: The Essential Guide to Loving Your Body Before and After Baby, by Claire Mysko, & Magali Amadeï

People might tell you you're glowing, but you just feel like you're growing, and perhaps you're not liking—or even recognizing—the changing image you see in the mirror. If you're like most expectant women, you're worried about what pregnancy and motherhood will do to your body, your sexuality, and your self-esteem.

Enter beauty activists Claire Mysko and Magali Amadei, who reveal a much-needed forewarning on what to expect from your changing body, as well as a reality check for each stage of your pregnancy. They expose the myths, challenges, and insecurities you'll face throughout pregnancy and beyond.

RECOMMENDED APPS

Pregnancy Tracker & Baby Development Calendar

From the brand chosen by over 400 million expecting parents, BabyCenter's pregnancy tracker and baby development calendar app for expecting moms will guide you through your pregnancy – week-by-week and day-by-day – with pregnancy tips and fetal development videos timed for your exact stage of pregnancy.

Join a community of other expectant moms and share your pregnancy experiences and struggles.
A great way to glean support when you're working on loving your pregnant body.

Hands Up Therapy

From an early age, society teaches us that some emotions are bad and should be avoided at all costs. As a result, we learn to avoid certain emotions, which can cause them to endure and mental health problems to arise. The Hands Up Therapy app teaches us how to stop avoiding emotions and deal with them in a healthy way, allowing us to achieve more peace and better mental health in the long run. The perfect companion for managing challenging emotions that arise when working on loving your pregnant body.

GADGETS AND PRODUCTS

Burt's Bees Mama Bee Belly Butter

Nourish your belly before and after pregnancy with this rich, moisturizing Burt's Bees Belly Butter that softens and smooths skin with a blend of naturally hydrating cocoa, shea and jojoba butters. Non-irritating and 99% natural formulated without phthalates, parabens, petrolatum, or SLS.

Designed specifically for mamas and mamas-to-be. A great product to help you show your pregnant body some love!

You're going to be the best mommy onesie

This cute one-piece baby bodysuit is perfect for your yet unborn little one! What a great reminder, even before the birth, that you are going to be the greatest mother to your child.

The Belly Book: A Nine-Month Journal for You and Your Growing Belly

Before you get to meet your baby, you spend a swell (so to speak) nine months getting acquainted with your growing belly. The first pregnancy journal devoted 100% to you and your belly, *The Belly Book* is organized by trimester and includes pages for "time-lapse" belly photos and ultrasound images, as well as prompts for writing about morning sickness, food cravings, maternity clothes you never want to see again, and much more.

A great companion to help you take loving your pregnant body to the next level.